PRESENT DAY PARKINSON'S DISEASE

Promotion of health, prevention and cure of Parkinson's Disease.

By Michael D. Hamilton

TABLE OF CONTENT

TABLE OF CONTENT

Disclaimer

The items in this book, wrote by Michael D. Hamilton, depend on the creator's exploration, encounters, and feelings. While each work has been made to give exact and exceptional data, readers are urged to freely check subtleties and look for proficient counsel if necessary. The writer and distributer renounce any risk or obligation regarding any misfortune, harm, or burden caused because of the utilization of data introduced in this book. Individual encounters might differ, and the book is certainly not a substitute for customized direction.

INTRODUCTION

In the domain of neurological issues, Parkinson's Sickness remains a considerable enemy, influencing millions around the world. As we explore the intricacies of the current day, it turns out to be progressively significant to unwind the secrets encompassing this condition. In "Present Day Parkinson's Illness," Michael D. Hamilton digs into the core of this mystery, offering perusers an adroit excursion through the contemporary scene of Parkinson's.

This extensive investigation isn't only a relating of side effects and clinical subtleties; it is a guide of understanding for patients, parental figures, and anybody contacted by the sweeping effect of Parkinson's. Hamilton's aptitude, established in both logical discernment and caring understanding, overcomes any issues between clinical talk and the human experience.

Perusers can anticipate a fastidiously created story that winds around together the logical progressions, individual tales, and cultural difficulties related to Parkinson's Infection. Hamilton's story voice reverberates with compassion, directing perusers through the many-sided trap of feelings that frequently go with a Parkinson's determination.

Besides, this book fills in as a significant asset for those looking for proactive measures against Parkinson's. Past revealing the complexities of the sickness, Hamilton frames down-to-earth procedures for avoidance, drawing upon the most recent exploration and leap forward. From the way of life acclimations to, rising clinical mediations, the writer engages perusers with information to face and alleviate the dangers related to Parkinson's.

Not halting at counteraction, Hamilton moves into the domain of possible fixes. Through an investigation of state-of-the-art medicines, exploratory treatments, and the most recent forward leaps in nervous system science, he paints a confident vision for a future where Parkinson's Sickness isn't recently overseen but won.

"Present Day Parkinson's Sickness" isn't simply a book; it's a demonstration of the strength of the human soul notwithstanding misfortune. Michael D. Hamilton welcomes perusers to leave on an excursion that joins logical thoroughness with caring narrating, cultivating a more profound comprehension of Parkinson's Infection and enlightening the way towards a more brilliant, better future.

Chapter 1.

Parkinson's illness: What is it, and what are the early signs?

An individual seeing a scarcely observable quake in one hand could be seeing the principal indications of Parkinson's illness.

This dynamic condition influences the sensory system, as per the Mayo Center in Rochester, Minn., which offers data about the illness.

While quakes are normal, Parkinson's can likewise cause solidness or sluggish development.

Drugs can fundamentally work on an individual's side effects. While the illness can't be restored, medical procedures might assist with managing specific districts of the mind and further develop side effects.

In the beginning phases, an individual's face might show practically no demeanor. Arms may not swing when somebody strolls. Talk could end up being sensitive or slurred. Side effects can deteriorate as the condition advances.

They frequently start on one side of the body. Commonly, they are more regrettable on that side, even after the condition starts influencing appendages on the two sides.

The Mayo Facility offers extra data on the exemplary side effects.

Quake, or cadenced shaking, regularly starts in the hand or fingers. An individual might rub their thumb and pointer to and fro. This is called a pill-moving shake.

The hand may likewise shudder when it's very still, yet that might diminish when an individual is tackling errands.

Another normal side effect is eased back development, additionally called bradykinesia. This is seen when straightforward errands become more troublesome: Steps might be more limited, it's hard to escape a seat, or there's hauling or rearranging feet while strolling.

Muscle firmness can happen in any piece of the body, may restrict the scope of movement, and can be difficult.

Stance might become stooped, and an individual with Parkinson's sickness might fall or have balance issues.

It might turn out to be harder to flicker, grin, or swing arms.

Discourse can likewise change, becoming gentler, faster, slurred, or reluctant. A droning might be created, as indicated by the Mayo Center.

Penmanship might seem more modest and it can become more earnest to compose.

It's essential to see a specialist on the off chance that you or a friend or family member has any of those side effects to get a finding or preclude different causes, as the Mayo Center desires.

What is the reason for Parkinson's infection?

There is nobody known reason for Parkinson's infection, however, there are factors that could increase risk. For most instances of the sickness, the reason is obscure.

An individual who is analyzed without cause has what is called an idiopathic Parkinson's infection.

The greatest gamble factor for Parkinson's sickness is age, as it is more considered normal seen in more established individuals. Orientation likewise assumes a part since guys are bound to get Parkinson's than females.

Rehashed head injury can build an individual's gamble, as could natural elements at any point like openness to pesticides and herbicides utilized for cultivating.

Chapter 2.

Reasons for Parkinson's illnesses

Specialists at the College of Helsinki have shown that specific types of Desulfovibrio microbes are the possible reason for Parkinson's sickness by and large. The review empowers the screening of the transporters of Desulfovibrio strains and the expulsion of the microscopic organisms from the stomach.

"Our discoveries are critical, as the reason for Parkinson's infection has gone obscure in spite of endeavors to recognize it over the past two centuries. The discoveries show that particular types of Desulfovibrio microorganisms are probably going to cause Parkinson's illness. The infection is fundamentally brought about by ecological elements, or at least, natural openness to the Desulfovibrio bacterial strains that cause Parkinson's sickness. Just a little offer, or generally 10%, of Parkinson's infection is brought about by individual qualities," says Teacher Per Saris from the College of Helsinki.

The objective of Teacher Saris' examination bunch was to tentatively explore whether the Desulfovibrio strains found in patients can bring about progress toward Parkinson's illness.

The chief finding of the gathering's late distributed study was that these strains in patients with Parkinson's illness cause a total of the α-synuclein protein on a genuinely critical level in a model living being for Parkinson's sickness. The worm Caenorhabditis elegans was utilized as the model life form.

The investigation additionally discovered that Desulfovibrio strains confined from sound people don't make α-synuclein total a similar degree. Conversely, the totals brought about by the Desulfovibrio strains in patients with Parkinson's sicknesses were likewise bigger.

"Our disclosures make it possible to assess for the carriers of these terrible Desulfovibrio microorganisms. Thus, they can be focused on by measures to eliminate these strains from the stomach, possibly mitigating and easing back the side effects of patients with Parkinson's sickness.

When the Desulfovibrio microorganisms are dispensed with from the stomach, α-synuclein totals are not generally shaped in that frame of mind, from which they travel towards the cerebrum through the vagus nerve-like prion proteins," Saris summarizes.

What Causes Parkinson's Sickness?

Parkinson's sickness is a persistent, moderate neurological illness that presently influences around 1 million Americans. Parkinson's sickness includes a little, dimly touched piece of the mind called the substantia nigra. This is where you produce the greater part of the dopamine your cerebrum utilizes. Dopamine is the synthetic courier that sends messages between nerves that control muscle development, as well as those engaged with the mind's pleasure and award, focuses. As we age, it's typical for cells in the substantia nigra to pass on. This cycle occurs in a great many people at an exceptionally sluggish rate.

However, for certain individuals, the misfortune happens quickly, which is the beginning of Parkinson's infection. At the point when 50 to 60 percent of the cells are gone, you start to see the side effects of Parkinson's.

Nobody Conclusive Reason for Parkinson's

There are no biomarkers or goal screening tests that show one has Parkinson's. All things considered, clinical specialists have shown that a star grouping of variables is connected to it.

Parkinson's causes are possibly a mix of hereditary qualities and ecological or other obscure variables. "Around 10 to 20 percent of Parkinson's illness cases are connected to a hereditary reason," says Ted Dawson, M.D., Ph.D., overseer of the Organization for Cell Designing at Johns Hopkins. The sorts are either autosomal prevailing (in which you get one duplicate of a transformed quality from one parent) or autosomal passive (in which you get a duplicate of a changed quality from every one of your folks).

However, that leaves most of Parkinson's cases as idiopathic, and that implies obscure. "We believe it's likely a blend of natural openness — to poisons or pesticides — and your hereditary cosmetics," says Dawson.

Age: The greatest gamble factor for fostering Parkinson's is propelling age.

Orientation: The typical time of beginning is 60. Men are bound to foster Parkinson's illness more than ladies.

Hereditary qualities: People with a parent or kin who are impacted have roughly twice the possibility of fostering Parkinson's. "There's been a colossal proportion of new information about inherited characteristics and new characteristics recognized over the past 10 or 15 years that have opened up a more unmistakable comprehension of the sickness," says Dawson.

Head injury. Rehashed hits to the head — think fighters, similar to Muhammad Ali — logically build one's gamble of fostering Parkinson's, however "Right now, we don't be aware with 100% conviction that it causes the infection," says Liana Rosenthal, M.D., partner teacher of nervous system science at the Johns Hopkins College Institute of Medication. "Only one out of every odd individual who gets head injury will encourage Parkinson's, and we can't 100%

guarantee that there's a sort, reality or repeat of head injury that extends your gamble."

Rest Unsettling influences

Tragically, rest unsettling influences are one of the most well-known non-engine side effects of Parkinson's Illness. Individuals with Parkinson's illness might encounter rest issues like distinctive dreams, bad dreams, and, surprisingly, carrying on dreams. These issues will more often than not progress with the illness. Parkinson's illness can disturb the cerebrum's regular rest wake cycle, which can cause these rest issues. There are various motivations behind why these rest issues occur, and scarcely any examinations have been finished to track down powerful medicines. All alone, rest aggravations are not a sign of Parkinson's sickness. Be that as it may, assuming you truly do end up with in excess of two or three of the side effects on this rundown, you ought to make a meeting with your medical services supplier.

Chapter 3

Side effects of parkinson's disease

Rest Aggravations:

Rest aggravations arc one of the most well-known non-engine side effects of Parkinson's Infection. Individuals with Parkinson's sickness might encounter rest issues like clear dreams, bad dreams, and, surprisingly, carrying on dreams. These issues will quite often advance with the sickness. Parkinson's infection can disturb the mind's normal rest wake cycle, which can cause these rest issues. There are various motivations behind why these rest issues occur, and scarcely any investigations have been finished to track down powerful medicines. All alone, rest aggravations are not a sign of Parkinson's infection. Be that as it may, assuming you really do wind up with in excess of two or three of the side effects on this rundown, you ought to make a meeting with your medical services supplier

Trouble Gulping:

Gulping troubles and slobbering are normal side effects that influence many individuals with Parkinson's sickness. These issues can prompt awkward and humiliating circumstances, as well as increase the gamble of pneumonia and different complexities. In Parkinson's sickness, the muscles in the mouth and throat can become feeble, making it hard to swallow food and drink. This can cause stifling, hacking, and trouble relaxing. Slobbering is additionally normal, as the muscles in the mouth and throat may not work as expected. There are various ways of dealing with these side effects, like changing the surface of food and beverages, taking prescriptions, and rehearsing activities to reinforce the muscles. Looking for the assistance of a language teacher or word-related specialist can likewise be valuable in improving gulping capability and diminishing slobbering.

Loss Of Smell (Anosmia):

Loss of smell, or anosmia, is a typical non-engine side effect of Parkinson's illness (PD). It can happen a very long time before engine side effects are created and is believed to be brought about by the degeneration of nerve cells in the olfactory framework. Research has shown that a deficiency of smell might be a helpful early marker for PD and that it is related to additional serious engine side effects and a more prominent mental degradation. While there is as of now no solution for anosmia in PD, studies have investigated the possible utilization of olfactory preparation and different medicines to assist with dealing with this side effect. Moreover, the exploration recommends that the utilization of olfactory testing can assist clinicians with diagnosing PD and screen the movement of the illness.

Stomach Issues and Parkinson's Sickness:

Clearly, stomach issues are not selective to Parkinson's sickness. Notwithstanding, this is a less popular issue that individuals experiencing the infection might have insight into. This study talks about the likely association between the stomach and the cerebrum in Parkinson's sickness and investigates the chance of utilizing food-based treatments to further develop side effects. It features the job of the stomach microbiome in the turn of events and movement of Parkinson's sickness, and looks at the effect of various dietary elements on the microbiome and what they might mean for the illness. The text proposes that a superior comprehension of the connection between the stomach and the mind, and the utilization of food-based treatments, may offer a promising way to deal with dealing with Parkinson's sickness.

Agony and Awareness:

One of the most troublesome side effects to make do with Parkinson's Sickness is the constant aggravation that most probably accompanies the analysis. The aggravation can take different structures, for example, outer muscle, dystonic, or neuropathic torment. Studies have shown that agony influences up to 85% of individuals with PD, and it can affect their personal satisfaction, mindset, and portability. The reasons for torment in PD are complicated and multifactorial, however, they might remember changes in the tactile handling and the focal aggravation adjustment framework. The article additionally examines the administration of torment in PD, which might include meds, non-intrusive treatment, workouts, and different medications.

Dystonia and Parkinson's Illness:

Agonizing constrictions, known as dystonia, can make life for Parkinson's Illness patients troublesome. Dystonia is a development problem that can happen in PD and other neurological circumstances. Dystonia is portrayed by compulsory muscle compressions that cause bending and dull developments or unusual stances. It can influence various pieces of the body, like the neck, face, arms, or legs, and it very well may agonize and cripple. The reasons for dystonia may include irregularities in the basal ganglia, a mind district that is impacted in PD. Conclusion and treatment of dystonia in PD might include drugs, botulinum poison infusions, profound mind feeling, or active recuperation.

Bladder and Gut Issues:

Parkinson's illness is brought about by the degeneration of nerve cells in a piece of the cerebrum called the substantia nigra. This prompts a decline in dopamine, a substance that assists with controlling development. Nonetheless, dopamine likewise assumes a part in managing the autonomic sensory system, which controls compulsory physical processes like bladder and gut control. Subsequently, individuals with Parkinson's sickness might encounter bladder and gut issues because of disturbances in this framework. Furthermore, the muscles that control these capabilities might become more fragile after some time, adding to challenges with urinary and inside self-restraint. These issues can be a wellspring of humiliation and inconvenience for those impacted, yet they can be dealt with with the right methodology. Treatment choices might incorporate medicine, pelvic floor activities, and dietary changes.

Discourse and Correspondence Hardships:

Parkinson's infection can influence development as well as discourse and gulping, which can essentially affect personal satisfaction. Perhaps the most detaching side effect of PD is discourse and correspondence issues. As the sickness advances, the muscles liable for discourse and gulping can become more fragile and less planned, prompting hardships with verbalization, voice projection, and eating. These side effects can be made with different treatments, like language instruction and dietary changes, as well as drugs that assist in further developing muscle control.

Orthostatic Hypotension:

Orthostatic hypotension is a typical issue experienced by individuals with Parkinson's illness. It is an unexpected drop in circulatory strain that happens while standing up from a sitting or lying position, which can cause tipiness, discombobulation, and in any event, swooning. This can be especially hazardous for people with Parkinson's sickness, who might be at an expanded gamble of falls and different wounds. Orthostatic hypotension can be made due to way of life changes like drinking more liquids, expanding salt admission, and staying away from unexpected changes. There are likewise drugs accessible that can assist with managing circulatory strain and further develop side effects.

Freezing of Stride:

Freezing of stride is a typical and baffling side effect of Parkinson's infection that influences portability and equilibrium. It happens when an individual out of nowhere feels like their feet adhere to the ground and they can't move forward. This can prompt falls and wounds, and can essentially influence an individual's personal satisfaction. The specific reason for freezing of step in Parkinson's illness isn't completely perceived. Notwithstanding, it is believed to be connected with the progressions in the mind that happen because of the sickness. Parkinson's sickness influences the dopamine-delivering cells in the mind, which assume an urgent part in managing development. As the sickness advances, these cells become harmed, prompting a decline in dopamine levels. This can cause a scope of engine side effects, including quakes, inflexibility, and trouble starting development, which can add to the freezing of walk. Also, freezing of stride can be set off by ecological factors like thin entryways, groups, or uneasiness.

A propensity to fidget:

Fretful leg disorder (RLS) is a typical condition that influences many individuals with Parkinson's sickness. It is portrayed by a mind-boggling desire to move the legs, which is many times joined by awkward sensations like shivering, copying, or creeping. RLS can cause critical rest aggravations, which can thus demolish different side effects of Parkinson's illness. At the point when dopamine levels are low, it can prompt a scope of engine side effects, including quakes and solidness, as well as non-engine side effects like rest unsettling influences, melancholy, and uneasiness. RLS might be connected with dopamine brokenness in the cerebrum, albeit the specific systems are not surely known. Also, RLS might be brought about by different factors like lack of iron, fringe neuropathy, or drugs used to treat Parkinson's illness.

Extreme Perspiring:

Extreme perspiring, otherwise called hyperhidrosis, is a typical issue experienced by individuals with Parkinson's illness. It tends to be brought about by a few elements, including prescription secondary effects, changes in the sensory system, and changes in the body's thermoregulatory framework. Unreasonable perspiring can be especially tricky for people with Parkinson's infection, as it can add to skin bothering, parchedness, and social shame. Treatment choices for unreasonable sweating are breathable dress, and utilizing antiperspirants. At times, prescription changes or careful intercessions might be fundamental. With the ideal administration, many individuals with Parkinson's illness can effectively oversee unnecessary perspiring and work on their personal satisfaction.

Vision Changes:

Visual side effects are normal in Parkinson's illness and can incorporate obscured vision, twofold vision, and trouble with profundity discernment. These side effects can be brought about by a few elements, remembering changes for the sensory system, drug secondary effects, and eye issues. Parkinson's sickness influences the cerebrum's capacity to handle visual data, which can. prompt hardships with visual discernment and handling. Moreover, a few prescriptions used to treat Parkinson's illness can cause obscured vision or dry eyes, which can deteriorate visual side effects. Eye issues like waterfalls, glaucoma, and macular degeneration are additionally more normal in people with Parkinson's illness. People with Parkinson's sickness must get normal eye tests and illuminate their medical services supplier in the event that they encounter any visual side effects. Treatment choices for visual side effects might incorporate prescription changes, vision treatment, or careful medications.

Skin Changes and Parkinson's Illness:

Changes in the skin are a typical and disturbing side effect experienced by individuals with Parkinson's illness. These progressions can incorporate dry skin, sleck skin, tingling, and changes in pigmentation. The specific reason for these skin changes isn't completely perceived, yet they are believed to be connected with changes in the sensory system and to prescription secondary effects. Parkinson's illness can influence the autonomic sensory system, which controls many physical processes including skin dampness and temperature guidelines. Furthermore, a few meds used to treat Parkinson's infection can cause skin changes or unfavorably susceptible responses. People with Parkinson's infection actually should illuminate their medical services supplier assuming they are encountering any skin changes, so they can get suitable consideration and backing. Treatment choices for skin changes might incorporate lotions, cured creams, and way of life changes, for example, keeping away from triggers.

Trouble with Fine Coordinated movements:

This is presumably the side effect that is generally usually connected with Parkinson's sickness. PD makes quakes due to the deficiency of dopamine-creating neurons in the cerebrum, explicitly in a space called the substantia nigra. Dopamine is a compound courier that directs development and coordination, and when there is an absence of dopamine, it prompts unusual action in the piece of the cerebrum that controls development. This unusual action can bring about quakes and other development issues that are normal for Parkinson's illness. The quakes in Parkinson's normally start in one hand or arm and can spread to different pieces of the body over the long run. While not all individuals with Parkinson's experience quakes, they are a typical side effect of the infection.

State of Mind and Conduct Changes:
Parkinson's illness isn't exclusively an actual sickness. It can likewise prompt conduct and mindset changes. These progressions can incorporate expanded uneasiness, crabbiness, and withdrawal from social circumstances, as well as trouble-controlling driving forces like betting or gorging. These non-engine side effects can fundamentally affect the personal satisfaction of individuals with Parkinson's. The deficiency of dopamine in the cerebrum and the utilization of specific meds to treat Parkinson's might add to these conduct changes. One more possible justification for these sorts of changes could be ascribed to the difficulties that PD patients face. It is insightful to counsel psychological medical care proficiently. This can assist in adapting to these troublesome life-altering events the side effects cause.

Motivation Control Issues:

This article from the American Parkinson's Illness Affiliation examines drive control issues (ICDs) in Parkinson's sickness. ICDs are a gathering of ways of behaving that incorporate impulsive betting, gorging, hypersexuality, and other exorbitant ways of behaving that can happen in individuals with Parkinson's who are being treated with dopamine agonist medicine. The article depicts the side effects of ICDs and what they can mean for an individual's life, as well as the gamble factors for creating ICDs. It likewise gives data on the most proficient method to oversee and treat ICDs in individuals with Parkinson's, including decreasing or changing dopamine agonist medicine and looking for guiding or other social treatments. The article stresses the significance of examining any progressions in conduct with a medical care supplier and cooperating to find the best therapy approach for the person.

Spit Creation:

Slobbering is a typical side effect of Parkinson's illness and happens because of changes in the muscles of the mouth and throat. Parkinson's can cause trouble gulping, diminished facial muscle control, and diminished spit control, all of which can add to slobbering. While slobbering can be humiliating and awkward, it is generally not a serious clinical issue. There are a few techniques that can help oversee slobbering in Parkinson's, for example, keeping up with great oral cleanliness, taking medicine to lessen spit creation, and rehearsing specific activities to reinforce the muscles in the mouth and throat.

Chapter 4.

Ways of forestalling Parkinson's sicknesses

Beginning around 2006, a few longitudinal investigations have surveyed natural or social factors that appear to change the gamble of fostering Parkinson's illness. Expanded hazard of Parkinson's sickness has been related to openness to pesticides, utilization of dairy items, history of melanoma, and horrendous cerebrum injury, while a decreased gamble has been accounted for in a relationship with smoking, caffeine utilization, higher serum urate focuses, actual work, and utilization of ibuprofen and other normal meds. Randomized preliminaries are researching the likelihood that a portion of the negative gamble variables may be neuroprotective and in this way gainful in people with early Parkinson's sickness, especially as for smoking (nicotine), caffeine, and urate. Later on, it very well may be feasible to recognize Parkinson's sickness in its prodromal stage and to advance neuroprotective mediations before the beginning of engine side effects. As of now, notwithstanding, the main mediation that appears to be legitimate for the essential counteraction of Parkinson's illness is the advancement of active work, which is probably going to be gainful for the avoidance of a few persistent sicknesses.

Customary treadmill exercise might help in forestalling Parkinson's illness, as per new exploration. These discoveries give desire to non-drug medicines, as actual work, to dial back the movement of the sickness.

As per analysts in Italy, taking part in escalated workouts, for example, everyday treadmill runs, can animate the development of mind-determined neurotrophic factor (BDNF). It is a protein basic for the endurance and development of mind neurons.

By advancing the soundness of neurons, BDNF improves the cerebrum's ability to revamp and adjust, which is significant for learning and memory. Also, BDNF supports decreasing the spread of obsessive alpha-synuclein totals, related to neurodegenerative issues like Parkinson's. These totals steadily debilitate neurons liable for engine control in unambiguous mind locales. By restricting their spread, coordinated abilities are less seriously impacted. Safeguarding indispensable neurons likewise keeps up with individuals' capacity to process and grasp visual data.

Schematic portrayal of the course of events of the exploratory systems. Chart of rats on a treadmill. A rundown of weeks in Roman numerals
Schematic portrayal of the timetable of the trial systems and the association of the exploratory gatherings. Rodents were infused with α-syn-PFFs or PBS at 2 to 90 days. A month after the infusion, rodents were isolated into two gatherings, stationary and dynamic. The dynamic creatures were signed up for the treadmill convention for quite some time. Inactive rodents were presented to an

exploratory contraption that was turned off. All exploratory gatherings were then exposed to conduct tests and utilized for immunofluorescence, electrophysiological, and other morphological investigations. IHC, immunohistochemistry. (credit: Calabresi et al. from Science Advances)

The exploration group noticed an expansion in BDNF levels in the minds of creatures with beginning phase Parkinson's illness after day-to-day treadmill practice for a very long time.

"We have found a never seen part, through which exercise acted first and foremost periods of the infection prompts beneficial effects on improvement control that could persevere after some time even subsequent to preparing is suspended," says Dr. Paolo Calabresi, comparing creator and nervous system science teacher at the Rome Grounds of the Catholic College of Holy Heart, in a media discharge.

Calabresi further recommends that recognizing new remedial targets and useful markers could help with creating non-drug medicines to supplement current medication treatments. Parkinson's illness is a neurological condition that influences equilibrium, and coordination, and can cause compulsory developments like solidness and shakily.

"Our assessment bunch is locked in with a clinical primer to test whether serious action can perceive new markers to screen the disorder development moving back in starting stage patients and the profile of the movement of the illness" adds Dr. Calabresi.

Almost 1,000,000 individuals in the US are living with Parkinson's illness. That number is supposed to ascend to 1.2 million by 2030.

As Parkinson's illness includes neuroinflammatory and neuroimmune parts in its beginning phases, the review will likewise investigate the job of glial cells, particular cells offering help to neurons, and their current circumstance. This examination intends to reveal the sub-atomic and cell systems basic the noticed advantages of activity.

Alzheimer's, downturn, and heftiness are sicknesses that might actually be forestalled, on the off chance that not treated, by the right equilibrium of microscopic organisms, growths, and infection that live normally in our guts - known as the "stomach microbiome".

Presently, Finnish researchers say they have observed that specific types of stomach microscopic organisms are likewise the reasonable justification for Parkinson's infection.

A typical age-related neurodegenerative issue, Parkinson's causes accidental or wild developments and influences exactly 8,000,000 individuals around the world. Be that as it may, in spite of over 200 years of exploration, its fundamental causes are not completely perceived. On account of microbiome research, be that as it may, the riddle has at long last been edified.

"Parkinson's is principally brought about by natural factors, or at least, ecological openness to the Desulfovibrio bacterial strains, and just a little offer, approximately 10%, is brought about by individual qualities," said Teacher Per Saris, lead specialist, from the College of Helsinki, in a proclamation.

Past examination by Saris' group had previously resolved that the Desulfovibrio (DSV) microscopic organisms - a sort of microbes that retains poisonous sulfate - were more common and bountiful in an amount in Parkison's illness patients, particularly those encountering more serious side effects when contrasted and solid people.

Be that as it may, it had not been explored the way in which the microorganisms assumed a part in the illness' turn of events.

In any case, the group's latest tests distributed in the logical diary Wilderness - which looked at waste examples from 10 Parkinson's patients and their sound life partners - have affirmed the speculation.

Saris' group found that DSV microorganisms upgrade the total of a neuronal protein called alpha-synuclein - a protein that is tracked down fundamentally in neurons in the cerebrum - which is a sign of the sickness.

New expectation as trial Alzheimer's medication seems to slow the deterioration of the illness by a third

Last year, a 72-year-old Scottish lady named Happiness Milne coincidentally gave a critical leap forward in the discovery of Parkinson's.

She had seen that her significant other's smell changed 12 years before his finding with Parkinson's, taking note that he had fostered a musky fragrance, not quite the same as his typical fragrance.

A group at the College of Manchester then saddled her power and found that Parkinson's sickness truly does without a doubt have a specific scent.

Furthermore, with Milne's assistance, they fostered a test that could decide in only three minutes whether somebody had the sickness.

Saris says Milne's revelation is lined up with his own group's disclosures.

There were two or three finds out about what mixtures were causing the smell and I checked if the Desulfovibrio minute living beings been able to convey these mixtures, and think about what was the outcome. Indeed, they can, nothing unexpected," he told Euronews Next.

A lady who can 'smell' Parkinson's illness assists researchers with creating a 3-minute skin swab test

For a really long time, patients and specialists have flagged digestive issues as a potential mark of Parkison's sickness.

"Individuals have revealed encountering clogging a long time before the side effects previously come in, and for quite a while, this has had individuals figuring there may be a poison or microbes that was starting the improvement towards Parkinson's sickness," Saris said.

His group's discoveries seem to affirm that hypothesis, while additionally giving an open door "to distinguish those with large quantities of microorganisms in their digestive tract, and afterward figure out who might be in danger of fostering Parkison's in ten or 20 years.

Saris likewise trusts specialists could direct screenings to distinguish the Parkinson-related microorganisms - and hence eliminate them from the stomach, "possibly mitigating and easing back the side effects of patients with Parkinson's sickness".

"We previously fostered a strategy to sort of effectively recognize on the off chance that you have a ton of Desulfovibrio in your defecation," he notes.

The first crap relocation treatment has been supported in the US. How does waste treatment function?

Where does the Desulfovibrio come from?

Numerous people have this strain in their stomach related organs," said Saris.

"It is in the climate, in the dirt, in the water, and furthermore in food varieties. We fundamentally eat them consistently, however, in ordinary circumstances, they don't develop to extremely big numbers. Likewise, in a typical circumstance, you have this nitrogen sulfide detoxification compound that will keep you sound".

Saris says they are as yet running tests to figure out which are the best food sources to repress the improvement of the Desulfovibrio strains. Be that as it may, he suggests "a more veggie lover-based diet, with a lot of fiber".

"It's realized that there is a relationship between meat utilization and Parkinson's illness," he noted.

The Finnish researcher likewise suggests keeping away from any way of behaving that causes a gamble of irritation in the digestive organs, "and that implies, if conceivable, no pressure," he says. "Be cherished and love someone, go into nature, be in touch with microorganisms in the woodland and in touch with creatures," he exhorts, guaranteeing that related to a decent eating regimen, "will assist the digestive system with staying away from a condition of irritation".

Chapter 5

Relieving Parkinson's infections

Parkinson's fix: Everyday pill could assist with keeping illness from creating
A day-to-day pill could hinder Parkinson's from creating and prompting quakes and firmness
Pexels
The day-to-day pill raises, expects a huge number of individuals in England living with the illness
An everyday pill could deflect Parkinson's from creating and prompting quakes and firmness, another investigation recommends.

Researchers are set to uncover new discoveries this week with their medication competitor that could prevent Parkinson's from advancing.

Suggested by following tests with mice and utilizing cells from individuals with the condition, the news raises expects a huge number of individuals in England living with the illness.

Presently there is no solution for Parkinson's and all current treatment is intended to ease the side effects.
Researchers are set to uncover new discoveries this week with their new medication candidatePexels

In the UK, around 145,000 individuals are living with Parkinson's and it is the quickest-developing neurological condition on the planet.
Estimates propose that somewhere in the range of 2020 and 2030 the quantity of cases will ascend by a fifth.
Biopharmaceutical organization, Samsara Therapeutics has fostered a treatment that takes a gander at supporting an interaction known as "autophagy".

Peter Hamley, the boss logical official at Samsara Therapeutics, said the examination has uncovered that by supporting autophagy, the poisonous protein is decreased and everything development and engine control is recaptured in the mice that were tried in the preliminary.

He said: "We think there is plausible of exchanging [Parkinson's], in spite of the way that in light of everything, it would end it."

The organization wants to send off its most memorable human preliminary not long from now as would be considered normal to occur in Holland.

Following the preliminaries, the medication would be on course to be delivered in around five or six years' time.

Hamley added: "This moment there are no drugs which actually altogether influence the condition and its development."

The organization is expecting to send off its most memorable human preliminary later this yearPexels

He likewise proposed that later on, there might be a possibility to utilize autophagy to broaden an individual's solid life expectancy.

He said: "My view is, the point at which we get a safeguarded drug accessible that we know prompts autophagy or other entrancing life expectancy frameworks, then, at that point, we can see that applying that to individuals who don't have a sickness, however, I believe that is quite far off."

It comes as a feature of a rush of interest in science that could be useful to individuals who live better for longer.

Innovation grandees including Amazon's Jeff Bezos, PayPal pioneer Peter Thiel, and Google organizer Larry Page all have put resources into life span organizations.

Home Famous people Back to the Future Star.

Michael J. Fox Given Privileged Oscar For Raising an Immense $1.5B for Parkinson's Sickness Exploration, Fox Commitments 'No Retreat. No Acquiescence' Till He Has a Fix
VIPs, Motion pictures, NEWS, OSCARS

Back to the Future Star Michael J. Fox Given Privileged Oscar For Raising a Huge $1.5B for Parkinson's Illness Exploration, Fox Commitments 'No Retreat. No Acquiescence' Till He Has a Fix

Michael J. Fox Given Privileged Oscar For Raising an Enormous $1.5B for Parkinson's Infection

In spite of the astonishing advancement in the field of medication at the turn of the twentieth hundred years, there's still no legitimate remedy for an illness as upsetting as Parkinson's among the numerous different sicknesses that plague mankind without a fix. Back To The Future star Michael J. Fox is one of the numerous sad people to have been determined to have this sickness.

Nonetheless, he's made a remarkable name for himself in the film business in light of the fact that all things considered, he's Marty McFly. He's likewise ensured that he's put all of the abundances that he got into great use, putting a colossal piece into researching and tracking down a remedy for the infection, and it's procured him a privileged Oscar!

A Short History Of Michael J. Fox's Battle Against Parkinson's

Michael J. Fox was at the highest point of the world when Back To What Was in Store was delivered, in the long run proceeding with the establishment and finishing up it with a third and last film in 1990.

He would then get projected in the rom-com Doc Hollywood, and as the shooting system began he would begin showing side effects of Parkinson's sickness. He in the end determined to have the sickness in 1991 (at 29 years old!) after the underlying side effects and was informed that he would need to carry his bursting acting vocation to a sad end in a couple of years.

Dazed by the news that was broken to him, the Youngster Wolf star would slip into the gloom, nursing it significantly more with weighty drinking.

Notwithstanding, he in the long run recovered and chose to enlighten the world regarding his lamentable finding, and to go above and beyond, he would effectively utilize his abundance and turned into a backer of examination on Parkinson's sickness. He later established The

Michael J. Fox Establishment with an end goal to assist with finding a remedy for what is still now a serious infection.

The Michael J. Fox Establishment has now brought more than $1.5 billion up in research reserves, genuinely a surprising accomplishment, and for his endeavors, Fox has procured himself a privileged Oscar.

Michael J. Fox Gets Privileged Oscar For Parkinson's Backing

Michael J. Fox, who has always lost an Oscar in spite of his splendid history as an entertainer, just got one for his endeavors in upholding as well as aiding raise assets for the examination in tracking down a remedy for Parkinson's sickness.

During the yearly Lead Representatives Grants service, Fox was given a wildly energetic applause by countless Elite entertainers in the group, like Tom Hanks and Jennifer Lawrence, as he acknowledged the Jean Hersholt Compassionate Honor. He also said

"It is lowering in the most profound manner to remain here and acknowledge your benevolence."

Taking everything into account, an Oscar for the Marty McFly entertainer was very much past due, yet it's ideal to commend the way that he authoritatively has one to his name now!

There's no solution for Parkinson's infection, now medicines are accessible to assist with letting the side effects and keeping up with your quality free from life.

These medicines include:

*steady treatments, like physiotherapy

*medicine

*medical procedure (for certain individuals)

You may not require any treatment during the beginning phases of Parkinson's infection as side effects are generally gentle.

However, you might require ordinary meetings with your subject matter expert so your condition can be observed.

You may be offered a gadget to wear at home that screens your side effects. The gadget imparts significant data to your trained professional.

A consideration plan ought to be concurred with your medical services group and your family or carers.

This will frame the medicines and assist you with requiring now and what you're probably going to require from now on, and ought to be surveyed consistently.

Strong treatments:

There are a few treatments that can make living with Parkinson's sickness more straightforward and assist you with managing your side effects on an everyday premise.

There are endeavors in progress to attempt to expand the accessibility of these steady treatments for Parkinson's patients on the NHS.

Your nearby authority might have the option to prompt and help you. Ask your nearby expert for a consideration and backing needs evaluation.

Physiotherapy:

A physiotherapist can work with you to ease muscle firmness and joint agony through development (control) and exercise.

The physiotherapist means to make moving more straightforward and work on your strolling and adaptability.

They likewise attempt to further develop your wellness levels and capacity to oversee things for yourself.

Word related treatment:

A word-related specialist can distinguish areas of trouble in your daily existence, like dressing yourself or getting to the nearby shops.

They can assist you with working out functional arrangements and guarantee your house is protected and appropriately set up for you. This will assist you with keeping up with your freedom as far as might be feasible.

Discourse and language treatment:

Many individuals with Parkinson's illness have gulping troubles (dysphagia) and issues with their discourse.

A discourse and language specialist can frequently assist you with working on these issues by showing talking and gulping works out, or by giving assistive innovation.

Diet counsel:

For certain individuals with Parkinson's sickness, rolling out dietary improvements can assist with working on certain side effects.

These progressions can include:

Expanding how much fiber in your eating routine and ensuring you're drinking sufficient liquid to diminish obstruction

expanding how much salt in your eating regimen and eating little, regular feasts to keep away from issues with low circulatory strain, for example, dazedness when you stand up rapidly

making changes to your eating routine to stay away from accidental weight reduction

You might see a dietitian, a medical services proficient prepared to offer eating regimen guidance, in the event that your consideration group figures you might profit from changing your eating routine.

Drug

Medicine can be utilized to work on the primary side effects of Parkinson's sickness, like shaking (quakes) and development issues.

In any case, not every one of the meds accessible is valuable for everybody, and the short- and haul impacts of each are unique.

Three fundamental kinds of medicine are ordinarily utilized:
*Levodopa
*Dopamine agonists
*Monoamine oxidase-B inhibitors

Your expert can make sense of your medicine choices, incorporating the dangers related to every drug, and talk about which might be best for you.
Standard surveys will be expected as the condition advances and your necessities change.

Levodopa:
The vast majority with Parkinson's infection in the long run need a drug called levodopa.

Levodopa is consumed by the nerve cells in your cerebrum and transformed into the substance dopamine, which is utilized to send messages between the pieces of the mind and nerves that control development.

Expanding the degrees of dopamine utilizing levodopa generally further develops development issues.

It's generally taken as a tablet or fluid and is frequently joined with other prescriptions, for example, benserazide or carbidopa.
These meds stop the levodopa from being separated in the circulatory system before it gets an opportunity to get to the cerebrum.
They likewise diminish the results of levodopa, which On the off chance that you're endorsed levodopa, the underlying portion is typically tiny and will be slowly expanded until it produces results.

From the start, levodopa can cause an emotional improvement in the side effects.

Be that as it may, its belongings can be less dependable throughout the next years - as more nerve cells in the mind are lost, there are fewer of them to retain the medication.
This implies the portion might be expanded occasionally.

Long-haul utilization of levodopa is likewise connected to issues like wild, jerky muscle developments (dyskinesias) and "on-off" impacts, where the individual quickly switches between having the option to continue (on) and being fixed (off).

Dopamine agonists:

Dopamine agonists go about as a substitute for dopamine in the cerebrum and have a comparative yet milder impact contrasted and levodopa. They can frequently be given less every now and again than levodopa.

They're many times taken as a tablet, but on the other hand, are accessible as a skin fix (rotigotine).

Once in a while, dopamine agonists are taken simultaneously as levodopa, as this permits lower dosages of levodopa to be utilized.

Conceivable symptoms of dopamine agonists include:

*Feeling and being debilitated
*Sluggishness and languor

*Unsteadiness

Dopamine agonists can likewise create pipedreams and expanded turmoil, so they should be utilized with an alert, especially in old patients, who are more defenseless.

For certain individuals, dopamine agonists have been connected to the improvement of habitual ways of behaving, particularly at high dosages, including habit-forming betting, urgent shopping, and an unnecessarily expanded interest in sex.

Converse with your medical services subject matter expert in the event that you figure you might be encountering these issues.

As the actual individual may not understand the issue, it's vital that carers and relatives likewise note any strange way of behaving and talk about it with a suitable expert at the earliest open door.

In the event that you're endorsed a course of dopamine agonists, the underlying portion is normally tiny to forestall feeling debilitated and opposite secondary effects.

The dose is continuously expanded north of half a month. On the off chance that feeling debilitated turns into an issue, your GP might endorse hostility to infection medicine.

A possibly serious, yet exceptional, intricacy of dopamine agonist treatment is the unexpected beginning of rest.

This by and large occurs as the portion is being expanded and will in general settle once the portion is steady.

Individuals are normally encouraged to abstain from driving while the portion is being expanded on the off chance that this complexity happens.

Monoamine oxidase-B inhibitors

Monoamine oxidase-B (MAO-B) inhibitors, including selegiline and rasagiline, are one more option in contrast to levodopa for treating early Parkinson's sickness.

They block the impacts of a compound or cerebrum substance that separates dopamine (monoamine oxidase-B), expanding dopamine levels.

Both selegiline and rasagiline can work on the side effects of Parkinson's infection, in spite of the fact that their belongings are little contrasted and levodopa. They can be utilized close by levodopa or dopamine agonists.

MAO-B inhibitors are for the most part all around endured, yet can sporadically cause incidental effects, including:

*Feeling wiped out

*Migraines

*Stomach torment

*High or low circulatory strain

Catechol-O-methyltransferase inhibitors

Catechol-O-methyltransferase (COMT) inhibitors are endorsed for individuals in later phases of Parkinson's sickness.

They forestall levodopa being separated by the catalyst COMT.

Symptoms of COMT inhibitors include:

*Feeling or being wiped out

*The runs

*tomach torment

*Non-oral treatments

At the point when Parkinson's side effects become challenging to control with tablets alone, various different medicines can be thought of.

Apomorphine

A dopamine agonist called apomorphine can be infused under the skin (subcutaneously) either by:

A solitary infusion, when required

A nonstop imbuement utilizing a little siphon hefted around on your belt, under your dress, or in a sack

Co-c carbidopa

For serious Parkinson's, a kind of levodopa called co-carbidopa might be siphoned persistently into your stomach through a cylinder embedded through your stomach wall.

There's an outer siphon appended to the furthest limit of the cylinder, which you haul around with you.

Some expert neuroscience places in the UK offer this treatment. It's just accessible assuming that you have extremely serious on-off variances or compulsory developments.

Parkinson's UK: imprudent and urgent ways of behaving in Parkinson's

Medical procedure

A great many people with Parkinson's illness are treated with medicine, albeit a kind of medical procedure called profound cerebrum excitement is utilized at times.

This medical procedure is likewise accessible in expert neuroscience revolves around the UK, however, it's not reasonable for everybody.

In the event that a medical procedure is being thought of, your expert will talk about the potential dangers and advantages with you.

Profound cerebrum feeling

Profound cerebrum feeling includes carefully embedding a heartbeat generator like a heart pacemaker into your chest wall.

This is associated with 1 or 2 fine wires set under the skin and is embedded exactly into explicit regions in your cerebrum.
A little electric momentum is created by the beat generator, which goes through the wire and invigorates the piece of your mind impacted by Parkinson's illness.

Despite the fact that medical procedure doesn't fix Parkinson's illness, it can facilitate the side effects for certain individuals.

Need to know more?

Decent: profound mind feeling for Parkinson's illness

Parkinson's UK: profound cerebrum feeling

Treating extra side effects

As well as the primary side effects of development issues, individuals with Parkinson's sickness can encounter a great many extra side effects that might be dealt with independently.
These include:

Melancholy and Nervousness - this can be treated by taking care of oneself through measures like activity, mental treatment or drug; read more about treating sorrow and treating tension

issues resting (a sleeping disorder) - this can be improved by making changes to your ordinary sleep time schedule; read more about treating sleep deprivation erectile brokenness - this can be treated with drugs; read more about treating erectile brokenness

extreme perspiring (hyperhidrosis) - this can be diminished by utilizing a remedy antiperspirant, or medical procedure in serious cases; read more about treating hyperhidrosis

gulping challenges (dysphagia) - this can be improved by eating mellowed food, or by utilizing a taking care cylinder in additional extreme cases; read more about treating dysphagia

unreasonable slobbering - this can be improved with gulping activities, medical procedures, or prescriptions in serious cases

urinary incontinence - this can be treated with activities to fortify the pelvic floor muscles, prescription, or medical procedure in serious cases; read more about treating urinary incontinence

dementia - this can be treated with mental treatments and prescription now and again; read more about treating dementia

Clinical preliminaries

Much headway has been made in the treatment of Parkinson's sickness as the consequence of clinical preliminaries, where new therapies and therapy blends are contrasted and standard ones.

All clinical preliminaries in the UK are cautiously managed to guarantee they're beneficial and securely directed. Members in clinical preliminaries now and again improve by and large than those in routine consideration.
If you've inquired as to whether you have any desire to partake in a preliminary, you'll be given a data sheet about the preliminary.
To participate, you'll be approached to sign an assent structure. You can decline to partake or pull out from a clinical preliminary without it influencing your consideration.

Need to know more?
Clinical preliminaries
Parkinson's UK: engage in research
Reciprocal and elective treatments
Certain individuals with Parkinson's illness find reciprocal treatments assist them with feeling far improved.

Numerous reciprocal medicines and treatments guarantee to facilitate the side effects of Parkinson's illness.

However, there's no clinical proof they're powerful at controlling the side effects of Parkinson's infection.

The vast majority think correlative medicines make no unsafe impacts. In any case, some can be destructive and ought not to be utilized rather than the drugs endorsed by your PCP.

A few kinds of homegrown cures, like St John's wort, can cooperate capriciously whenever taken for certain sorts of medicine used to treat Parkinson's infection.

Assuming you're thinking about utilizing an elective treatment alongside your endorsed drugs, check with your consideration group first.

Chapter 6

Logical forward leap of Parkinson's illnesses

The new remedial objective for Parkinson's illness found

Reestablishing contacts among mitochondria and lysosomes works on neuronal capability

Northwestern Medication researchers have revealed another system by which transformations in quality parkin add to familial types of Parkinson's illness. The revelation opens another road for Parkinson's therapeutics, researchers report in another review.

The Northwestern researchers found that changes in parkin bring about a breakdown of contacts between two vital laborers in the phone — lysosomes and mitochondria.

Mitochondria are the principal makers of energy in cells, and lysosomes reuse cell flotsam and jetsam that aggregate during the typical capability of our phones. These organelles are particularly significant in our minds since neurons are profoundly subject to energy creation by mitochondria, and in light of their movement, neurons produce an overflow of cell trash that should be cleared by lysosomes.

In an earlier report, distributed in Nature, Dr. Dimitri Krainc, seat of nervous system science and overseer of Simpson Querrey Community for Neurogenetics at Northwestern College Feinberg Institute of Medication, and his gathering found that lysosomes and mitochondria structure contacts with one another. After the underlying disclosure, Northwestern researchers attempted to grasp the capability of these contacts in Parkinson's sickness.

In the new review distributed July 19 in Science Advances, the specialists report that lysosomes help mitochondria by giving key metabolites their capability. Mitochondria should import a significant number of their fundamental fixings, however, it has not been notable where a portion of these metabolites come from. Then again, lysosomes act as reusing plants in cells and, thus, produce numerous breakdown items that could be utilized by different organelles, for example, mitochondria.

In this work, researchers found that lysosomes give significant amino acids that help the capability of mitochondria. In any case, they likewise found that in certain types of Parkinson's illness, lysosomes can't act as "some assistance" to mitochondria in light of the fact that the contacts between the two organelles are disturbed. This outcome in useless mitochondria and at last degeneration of weak neurons in Parkinson's sickness.

"Discoveries from this study propose that dysregulation of mitochondria-lysosome contacts adds to the Parkinson's infection pathophysiology," said Krainc, the review's comparing creator. "We recommend that reestablishing such mitochondria-lysosome contacts addresses a significant new helpful chance for Parkinson's infection."

According to a more extensive viewpoint, this study opens another road of examination in neurodegenerative problems, by featuring the significance of direct correspondence and coordinated effort between cell organelles in the pathogenesis of these issues.

Parkinson's Sickness: 5 Purposes Behind Trust

Doubtlessly a finding of Parkinson's is extraordinary and life-changing — yet it's not the demise of life as far as you might be concerned. Patients with Parkinson's have many motivations to be confident, from state-of-the-art exploration to better schooling that can assist you with remaining in control.

The following are five, just to give some examples.

Reason 1: Better, Longer Life Expectancies: Individuals with Parkinson's are living longer — yet in addition better. "We are getting better at dealing with the inconveniences of the infection. Patients are living longer and better than previously, even with practically no prescription," says Liana Rosenthal, M.D., collaborator teacher of nervous system science at the Johns Hopkins College Institute of Medication.

Reason 2: Prior Analysis: The sooner Parkinson's sickness can be distinguished, the more successfully it may be dealt with. Endeavors to focus in on the illness in prior stages are continuous, however, at this moment it's actually thought to be a "clinical finding," says Rosenthal. "That implies there is no blood or imaging test that can perceive us without a doubt that you have Parkinson's." Scientists are taking a gander at ways of pinpointing trademarks or side effects in prior stages. For instance, researchers in Britain have fostered a harmless eye test that can recognize Parkinson's before actual side effects are available. Noticing changes in the retina might offer signs.

Reason 3: State of the art Lab Exploration: At Johns Hopkins, an examination into the cooperation of qualities connected to Parkinson's infection might propose new and better treatment choices. For instance, the continuous investigation into how the Parkinson's sickness quality LRRK2 (likewise called LARK2) collaborates with other Parkinson's qualities is prompting a superior comprehension of how the illness advances — and how it very well may be eased back.

Reason 4: Clinical Preliminaries: Similarly as with any infection, clinical preliminaries offer scientists potential chances to track down better ways of identifying, overseeing, and dealing with sicknesses like Parkinson's. In any case, preliminaries are likewise an extraordinary chance for you, as a Parkinson's patient, to help with the disclosure of medicines. In 1997, the Public Foundation of Neurological Issues and Stroke (NINDS, part of the Public Organizations of Wellbeing) laid out the NINDS Morris K. Udall Focuses of Greatness for Parkinson's Infection Exploration program at Johns Hopkins.

Reason 5: High-level Medicines: One promising treatment is profound cerebrum feeling or DBS. This type of treatment involves electrical excitement in the cerebrum to treat Parkinson 's-related development issues, like quakes, solidness, trouble in strolling, and eased back development, and might be a choice when drugs become less powerful or aftereffects excessively difficult.

In a subsidized report by NINDS and the Division of Veterans Undertakings, DBS — when contrasted with drug and exercise-based recuperation for Parkinson's side effects — was predominant in working on engine side effects and personal satisfaction.

www.ingramcontent.com/pod-product-compliance
Lightning Source LLC
Chambersburg PA
CBHW050851260726
48660CB00006B/2561